Words can be found in all d...

- ☐ WELCOME
- ☐ CONGRATULATIONS
- ☐ WITH
- ☐ THIS
- ☐ SUPERHUGE
- ☐ FONT
- ☐ WORDSEARCH
- ☐ BOOK
- ☐ HAVE
- ☐ FUN

```
U D W O R D S E A R C H A V E
T X N S B M N A P K E C T J Y
H U X Y H W A Y R M X O U I X
I L B P D Y S S F W Z F M A W
S C G A W M E D I U M B D Y G
Y T L U C I F F I D N F O N T
S N O I T A L U T A R G N O C
E E G U H R E P U S W G E B K
X P K M W E L C O M E I Z M E
```

NAME: AGE:

THIS BOOK IS FOR PEOPLE WITH POOR EYESIGHT, OR ARTHRITIS. THESE WORD SEARCH LETTERS ARE NOT JUST BIG, BUT SUPERSIZED. GOOD LUCK!

When I created this book, I decided to not include the answers. Come on, you're a pro! Besides, this way we have more pages, so I can add more puzzles...

Nature edition

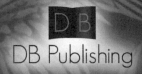

DB Publishing

VOL. 03

```
S X Q W N O R C H I D F F
A I N O C I L E H H H Q O
P N V K A P O K B H F H
B P B Q C B I A A B E C
H B A N A N A S G T U Q
E G V C O T N M S J Y R
D A I L E M O R B J A N
T A L F H I X P E O Q V
H B N Z N B B C F F O T
Z F M A H O G A N Y P D
M H I B I S C U S T X B
V A N I L L A Y R S T G
```

- BAMBOO
- BANANAS
- BROMELIAD
- CACAO
- CEIBA
- FERN
- FIG
- HELICONIA
- HIBISCUS
- KAPOK
- LIANA
- MAHOGANY
- ORCHID
- RUBBER
- VANILLA

```
Y M G Z A I C A C A C A E M
O I A B U S F S F S E N N A
K W E I H G L U P I N N N
S R E N N T D A V A U G
G A R J I O N B B Y B O
W E C S N P G A I B R Y
V I E C S A U E R Q M N
P K F D U E T L B A L G
N V N X Z Y R T A M M Q
P O T H O S C P A L M A
Z Y N T O N F A Y R G I
Z M A R A N T A T C K M
```

- [ ] ACACIA
- [ ] AMARANTH
- [ ] BALSA
- [ ] BEGONIA
- [ ] CYPRESS
- [ ] GUAVA
- [ ] LUPIN
- [ ] LUPINE
- [ ] MANGO
- [ ] MARANTA
- [ ] PALM
- [ ] POTHOS
- [ ] RATTAN
- [ ] SENNA
- [ ] YUCCA

3

```
P R K O T I U Q S O M V
W Q E W A S P F L Y H D
T E A P Z E E B I A L W
L D G T P C L L I T S U
O H N L E O I F T B Z K
C M A A W R H C C E P C
U W T N B E M S A Y E C
S K H T O M S I S D U B
T Q G E M Q D U T A A X
K R E R W B U P O E R X
W J U N E M F K V L M G
E U T H W K L I V E E W
```

☐ BEE   ☐ GNAT   ☐ MOSQUITO
☐ BEETLE   ☐ GRASSHOPPER ☐ MOTH
☐ CICADA   ☐ LANTERN   ☐ TERMITE
☐ FLEA   ☐ LOCUST   ☐ WASP
☐ FLY   ☐ LOUSE   ☐ WEEVIL

```
D X E D D P R J T Z Z T
R P G L L T I E Q O D H
A C H I G G E R D Q N R
G Z B H W Y D K H I A I
O I U M X R L I C T P P
N A T C O G A F T I O S
F U T V H S U E E N R S
L T E N G Q A B L R A C
Y I R G A P H I D C I M
U B F C B W B O R E R F
R Y L F Y A M J R C B R
G D Y Y B H A O J W J R
```

- ☐ ANT
- ☐ APHID
- ☐ BEDBUG
- ☐ BORER
- ☐ BUTTERFLY
- ☐ CHIGGER
- ☐ CRICKET
- ☐ DRAGONFLY
- ☐ EARWIG
- ☐ FIREFLY
- ☐ MANTID
- ☐ MAYFLY
- ☐ SPIDER
- ☐ THRIP
- ☐ THRIPS

```
C Q Y L E R R I U Q S O
A R M A D I L L O I M P
P B K G G N I R A M A T
U Y E O T R T W E R H S
C Y B U Y E A E T W E L
H U W T V M S M N H Y O
I O F I E A T O G R L T
N O W T T N B N M Q E H
X N L X P A C A U R W C
I P N Q W T O T I K A S
W P V I X E L C T C D M
X M E O C E L O T R C M
```

- AGOUTI
- ARMADILLO
- CAPUCHIN
- COATI
- MANATEE
- MARGAY
- MARMOSET
- OCELOT
- PACA
- SAKI
- SHREW
- SLOTH
- SQUIRREL
- TAMARIN
- TENREC

T	L	N	S	C	N	W	O	X	K	R	R
F	E	R	D	E	T	O	E	L	X	I	E
X	E	V	U	H	S	A	K	A	K	I	P
U	G	N	I	M	Y	O	R	A	S	V	R
I	O	N	W	C	E	R	O	S	N	E	W
U	P	J	O	G	A	L	A	G	I	V	L
I	I	A	A	R	J	B	Y	X	N	E	R
T	M	Q	K	K	U	E	Q	Z	A	O	R
E	O	J	U	O	N	T	R	W	U	W	M
E	L	O	V	D	C	I	N	B	Y	Q	V
L	E	R	U	F	U	Y	K	I	O	E	N
G	T	D	Z	I	I	P	Y	Z	B	A	J

- ☐ BINTURONG
- ☐ CIVET
- ☐ GALAGO
- ☐ HYRAX
- ☐ JERBOA
- ☐ KINKAJOU
- ☐ LEMUR
- ☐ MOLE
- ☐ MONGOOSE
- ☐ OKAPI
- ☐ PIKA
- ☐ PUDU
- ☐ TARSIER
- ☐ VOLE
- ☐ WEASEL

```
C O N D O R T E M C H K
K J Q M I X N O G O R T
E T Y T O L F H U R Q K
T C J T R T E E C C U I
Q O W C N Z M R G N A M
E G R E T H A O T X I N
H H C R Z Y C N T S L F
Q B I D A I A A A K E G
L Y Z D F P W S R C B K
E L O I R O S M I D A Y
O T M N G V O A C B G J
L T I B N U S L N H I X
```

☐ **CONDOR**　　☐ **JACANA**　　☐ **PARROT**
☐ **EGRET**　　　☐ **KESTREL**　 ☐ **QUAIL**
☐ **FINCH**　　　☐ **MACAW**　　 ☐ **SUNBIT**
☐ **HERON**　　　☐ **MOTMOT**　　☐ **TOUCAN**
☐ **IBIS**　　　　☐ **ORIOLE**　　☐ **TROGON**

```
H O N I K A N A M A M A U M
C O O R Q L N I P Y T L
T P I G E O N O F P M K
N H C I R T S O C F N D
W O S S A C T E Z L U P
U G Z E C O T I N G A P
B V A A J D S Y B A A F
W S M O M F U P O N R O
D R I B Y A J H R T R C
G R A L O R I K E E T I
Y V N A C I L E P M Y Z
W D D R O L L E R D O K
```

- AMAZON
- BITTERN
- CASSOW
- COTINGA
- CRANE
- FALCON
- JAYBIRD
- LORIKEET
- MANAKIN
- OSPREY
- OSTRICH
- PELICAN
- PIGEON
- PUFFIN
- ROLLER

```
Y U F F A I L L E M A C
E M V X X I W R O S E Z
L Y P P O P N A Z T I J
V D Y D N R A O P Y L Q
H I A X P J C E G H J J
A H Y H H E P H L E Q M
Y S A S L T O I I A B O
S C T M I I E N L D Z T
M T A E L A A L Y U E A
T V J L R D D U O M T Q
X L K X I A I N N I Z K
F Y U V T L P U N A V L
```

- [ ] ASTER
- [ ] AZALEA
- [ ] BEGONIA
- [ ] CAMELLIA
- [ ] DAHLIA
- [ ] DAISY
- [ ] LILAC
- [ ] LILY
- [ ] ORCHID
- [ ] PEONY
- [ ] POPPY
- [ ] ROSE
- [ ] TULIP
- [ ] VIOLET
- [ ] ZINNIA

```
Y H K C O H Y L L O H Y
L Y R P A N S Y G X Y J
L L D E K Y L I A O A A
S I E L S S E Q R S C S
U C D B O O A I D I I M
N V R O E G R T E X N I
F E H O F U I M N D T N
L R K F C F L R I O H E
O B Z M T U A B A R D B
W E T R G B S D J M P Q
E N U H E A T H E R V D
R A H M F A I S E E R F
```

- [ ] **BLUEBELL**
- [ ] **CROCUS**
- [ ] **DAFFODIL**
- [ ] **FREESIA**
- [ ] **GARDENIA**
- [ ] **HEATHER**
- [ ] **HOLLYHOCK**
- [ ] **HYACINTH**
- [ ] **IRIS**
- [ ] **JASMINE**
- [ ] **MARIGOLD**
- [ ] **PANSY**
- [ ] **PRIMROSE**
- [ ] **SUNFLOWER**
- [ ] **VERBENA**

```
N T L O B E L I A M W Z
X X O F W A E P T E E W S
J G G U M A I N U T E P
X T A A T U X I D H P Y
X O P N R Y I Z A K H A
D Q L E E D D N F X N R
S A A H N M P N A M E R
A O S R P I O A A R M O
L N M O R L P N N C E W
V U X S M O D U E S S G
I S U L O I D A L G I Q
A C Z W H C M P U J A G
```

- ANEMONE
- CANDYTUFT
- COSMOS
- GERANIUM
- GLADIOLUS
- LOBELIA
- LUPINE
- MIMOSA
- NEMESIA
- PETUNIA
- PHLOX
- SALVIA
- SNAPDRAGON
- SWEETPEA
- YARROW

```
M U M R E P S O E T S O
E N H B A I R E T S I W
K A L A N C H O E L A J
V S I L L Y R A M A H H
F T N S A X Y Y E N E B
G U A E H T P J J T L V
E R C G I C N E Q A E E
R T F R S T U A W N N R
B I E K F T A F R A I B
E U D A E R I P S A U E
R M W O R R A Y M P M N
A I N O H T I T H I J A
```

- [ ] AMARYLLIS
- [ ] FUCHSIA
- [ ] GERBERA
- [ ] HELENIUM
- [ ] IMPATIENS
- [ ] KALANCHOE
- [ ] LANTANA
- [ ] MARANTA
- [ ] NASTURTIUM
- [ ] OSTEOSPERMUM
- [ ] SPIREA
- [ ] TITHONIA
- [ ] VERBENA
- [ ] WISTERIA
- [ ] YARROW

D	Q	F	P	V	N	A	C	I	L	E	P
N	Z	F	A	O	B	X	C	B	N	O	T
K	H	A	T	L	G	M	L	I	I	H	F
D	R	E	L	O	C	N	L	S	E	Y	V
T	K	O	R	B	R	O	I	L	P	W	W
O	W	Z	T	O	A	R	N	M	U	B	O
E	I	N	Z	S	N	T	A	M	A	G	W
L	K	C	U	M	E	S	R	P	R	L	X
U	K	C	W	R	O	D	N	O	C	W	F
Y	I	S	I	H	C	I	R	T	S	O	U
B	U	T	V	U	L	T	U	R	E	S	L
H	X	V	W	P	E	A	C	O	C	K	U

☐ ALBATROSS ☐ FLAMINGO ☐ PARROT
☐ CONDOR ☐ GULL ☐ PEACOCK
☐ CRANE ☐ HERON ☐ PELICAN
☐ EMU ☐ IBIS ☐ STORK
☐ FALCON ☐ OSTRICH ☐ VULTURE

```
P W B P L O S P R E Y E
N R E T T I B B S A M C
E I P L L I B N O O P S
D R I B G N I M M U H A
S G G J H A R A V E N U
H A R P Y O E V D V W W
X N H E H U R I B A J T
V N H G P P E N Q I H P
R E D R A Z Z U B Z E T
Z T K E S T R E L I S H
O Y L T Y E K R U T L L
M V T N A S A E H P O L
```

- BITTERN
- BUZZARD
- EAGLE
- EGRET
- GANNET
- HARPY
- HORNBILL
- HUMMINGBIRD
- JABIRU
- KESTREL
- OSPREY
- PHEASANT
- RAVEN
- SPOONBILL
- TURKEY

J Q Y L N R E T C J S N
N M M A K I W I F R L P
G S E P J B U A Y H D Y
L W Y S Q I N G C E S O
O A G O K C T O N A X U
F N N R P I H G E E M N
S R J A O L M Z M G P U
E O L K C U D M Z Q I N
N O M S Q A S U E G C P
U K I T E X J E Y R X I
U H W X X B R L I A U Q
L U O O I M N Z T A O U

☐ **DUCK**
☐ **GROUSE**
☐ **JACANA**
☐ **JAY**
☐ **KITE**

☐ **KIWI**
☐ **MACAW**
☐ **PENGUIN**
☐ **PIGEON**
☐ **QUAIL**

☐ **RHEA**
☐ **ROOK**
☐ **SKIMMER**
☐ **SWAN**
☐ **TERN**

B	N	F	O	L	W	S	Y	S	T	J	O
J	X	T	C	O	T	V	M	M	S	F	R
H	Y	B	O	O	B	I	V	W	Q	E	I
G	C	P	J	N	O	Y	W	Y	B	F	O
T	A	N	T	R	A	T	S	D	E	R	L
W	O	L	I	I	U	G	K	W	O	I	E
P	E	M	L	F	N	G	B	L	Q	G	J
E	B	L	T	I	N	I	K	A	N	A	M
T	J	S	R	O	N	Z	F	P	H	T	K
R	I	H	H	U	M	U	P	F	B	E	F
E	S	Z	I	V	C	O	L	A	U	W	C
L	U	Q	H	O	O	P	O	E	O	P	B

☐ BOOBY ☐ GALLINULE ☐ MOTMOT

☐ COOT ☐ GODWIT ☐ ORIOLE

☐ CURLEW ☐ HOOPOE ☐ PETREL

☐ FINCH ☐ LOON ☐ PUFFIN

☐ FRIGATE ☐ MANAKIN ☐ REDSTART

```
S T U R G E O N L K K B
N T X G N O I L   A E S
A A A   J Q L C G J I D T
P R D D H N A T W F V B
P P E O U S I H O B T R
E O Z P L C I L W P J M
R N X D U P A F R R U B
M N W O Z O H R T A A S
S U R L A W R I R A M N
E H S I F L E G N A C Y
U L P H S I F E U L B X
B S A I L F I S H J S D
```

- [ ] **ANGELFISH**
- [ ] **BARRACUDA**
- [ ] **BLUEFISH**
- [ ] **CATFISH**
- [ ] **DOLPHIN**
- [ ] **GROUPER**
- [ ] **MARLIN**
- [ ] **NARWHAL**
- [ ] **OCTOPUS**
- [ ] **SAILFISH**
- [ ] **SEA LION**
- [ ] **SNAPPER**
- [ ] **STURGEON**
- [ ] **TARPON**
- [ ] **WALRUS**

```
G S T I N G R A Y Z W T
S U N F I S H B C X Z Y
K M E B E L U G A R M Z
O S W O R D F I S H U Y
B E A N U T P C H Y V X
T U B I L A H R G X K T
L E V T E S I O P R O P
Z M D O E E T A N A M O
S J Y L E R E K C A M F
J F L O U N D E R T Z H
W A H O O H E R R I N G
O J E L L Y F I S H V D
```

- BELUGA
- BONITO
- CROAKER
- FLOUNDER
- HALIBUT
- HERRING
- JELLYFISH
- MACKEREL
- MANATEE
- PORPOISE
- STINGRAY
- SUNFISH
- SWORDFISH
- TUNA
- WAHOO

```
W F G R E P P A N S R Q
O L S N D O D U P S O H
B A N K I W Z W A O Y A
B M H S I F D O C C N D
E P N K W C E G R J R D
G R I V R R A U H H R O
O E H T N A C A L E O C
N Y O H M Y H V X B E K
G C U Q V F S S I R I L
J E I H S I F R A O D A
D O G F I S H C R F U F
G N I T I H W Y A R O M
```

- ☐ BLUEFIN
- ☐ CODFISH
- ☐ COELACANTH
- ☐ CRAYFISH
- ☐ DOGFISH
- ☐ EEL
- ☐ HADDOCK
- ☐ LAMPREY
- ☐ MORAY
- ☐ OARFISH
- ☐ ORCA
- ☐ SHARK
- ☐ SNAPPER
- ☐ WHITING
- ☐ WOBBEGONG

R	S	A	R	G	A	S	S	U	M	H	J
T	E	O	N	B	V	W	R	A	S	S	E
R	W	H	S	I	F	R	A	G	V	N	S
E	H	L	R	F	V	A	T	L	C	B	T
V	A	P	R	K	Q	R	O	R	O	Q	L
A	L	E	P	O	L	L	O	C	K	M	H
L	E	R	H	S	I	F	K	C	O	R	V
L	F	C	F	N	T	A	R	P	O	N	I
Y	I	H	S	I	F	T	O	R	R	A	P
H	S	I	F	N	O	I	P	R	O	C	S
U	H	B	N	I	F	W	O	L	L	E	Y
E	S	S	A	B	A	E	S	H	J	A	R

- ☐ CORVINA
- ☐ GARFISH
- ☐ MOLA
- ☐ PARROTFISH
- ☐ PERCH
- ☐ POLLOCK
- ☐ ROCKFISH
- ☐ SARGASSUM
- ☐ SCORPIONFISH
- ☐ SEABASS
- ☐ TARPON
- ☐ TREVALLY
- ☐ WHALEFISH
- ☐ WRASSE
- ☐ YELLOWFIN

O	R	M	D	E	A	L	L	I	R	O	G
J	O	O	W	S	L	E	O	P	A	R	D
A	T	R	T	Y	A	A	W	B	I	H	Y
G	N	A	A	A	F	Q	K	U	C	I	R
U	G	T	R	G	G	V	C	F	H	N	C
A	T	A	E	E	N	I	Z	F	E	O	H
R	V	X	Z	L	F	A	L	A	E	C	Z
B	S	A	L	E	O	F	K	L	T	E	E
I	R	F	G	O	L	P	A	O	A	R	B
T	N	A	H	P	E	L	E	R	H	O	R
R	E	H	T	N	A	P	E	P	I	S	A
E	L	I	D	O	C	O	R	C	X	G	S

- [ ] ALLIGATOR
- [ ] ANTELOPE
- [ ] BUFFALO
- [ ] CHEETAH
- [ ] CROCODILE
- [ ] ELEPHANT
- [ ] GAZELLE
- [ ] GIRAFFE
- [ ] GORILLA
- [ ] JAGUAR
- [ ] KANGAROO
- [ ] LEOPARD
- [ ] PANTHER
- [ ] RHINOCEROS
- [ ] ZEBRAS

W	I	C	C	I	Q	L	L	E	P	A	P
I	V	M	D	O	N	K	E	Y	L	Z	X
L	J	I	P	D	K	D	A	R	X	E	R
D	E	L	B	A	S	A	F	Y	L	P	X
E	Q	P	W	X	L	U	P	J	A	N	M
B	L	E	M	A	C	A	R	I	B	O	U
E	W	U	P	N	U	K	M	L	E	M	S
E	J	W	J	W	N	B	R	A	A	V	T
S	Z	B	O	N	G	O	F	D	L	W	R
T	T	K	P	H	T	A	S	B	R	L	R
I	X	T	A	P	I	R	P	I	W	R	G
O	D	G	O	H	T	R	A	W	B	G	B

☐ BISON ☐ DONKEY ☐ TAPIR
☐ BOAR ☐ IMPALA ☐ WALRUS
☐ BONGO ☐ LLAMA ☐ WARTHOG
☐ CAMEL ☐ OKAPI ☐ WILDEBEEST
☐ CARIBOU ☐ SABLE ☐ YAK

```
N U D U K O S T R I C H
N I K A T R E V A E B S
O N V R D T A S Q S W J
P A A T W N H V O X H O
G J N T F B O F D O L R
F J V E U N B C W R M Y
P R X Z Y G O V A S A X
D M A W B H N H I N N A
I N I D H X N A T B A I
A H O H Z T K L R Y E Q
J H I I C G C H A O P X
F J A Y L Y E K N O M Z
```

- [ ] AARDVARK
- [ ] ANACONDA
- [ ] BEAVER
- [ ] CHIMP
- [ ] HYENA
- [ ] IBEX
- [ ] KUDU
- [ ] LION
- [ ] MONKEY
- [ ] MOOSE
- [ ] ORANGUTAN
- [ ] ORYX
- [ ] OSTRICH
- [ ] PYTHON
- [ ] TAKIN

W	D	E	M	K	B	E	O	E	Q	N	X
O	U	X	N	P	O	B	M	R	L	E	J
M	C	J	D	Y	R	A	G	U	O	C	P
B	H	O	G	N	I	D	L	L	W	V	P
A	E	L	Y	D	B	G	F	A	W	R	W
T	D	T	L	O	G	E	V	P	G	R	N
C	G	K	O	I	T	R	A	U	G	A	J
C	E	Q	N	L	R	E	E	R	Y	C	E
B	H	T	O	P	E	D	N	E	B	C	O
B	O	D	Y	T	F	C	N	M	D	O	K
Y	G	I	T	D	J	F	O	A	P	O	Y
N	E	V	O	H	T	O	L	S	M	N	G

- ☐ BADGER
- ☐ BEAR
- ☐ COUGAR
- ☐ COYOTE
- ☐ DEER
- ☐ DINGO
- ☐ EMU
- ☐ HEDGEHOG
- ☐ JAGUAR
- ☐ KOALA
- ☐ MANDRILL
- ☐ OCELOT
- ☐ RACCOON
- ☐ SLOTH
- ☐ WOMBAT

25

```
N O M M I S R E P B G Y
R S A V O K L E Z A J E
X L A I L O N G A M G L
S W C R U H I O W B C L
H I I U F E D L T O W O
E S T Q J A A Y X O A W
M T R I B E S A V O F W
L E U E B U J S W E Y O
O R S O D Q D V A T Q O
C I W I L L O W Z S I D
K A C A C I A S O M I M
S E R V I C E B E R R Y
```

- ACACIA
- ALDER
- BAMBOO
- CITRUS
- HEMLOCK
- MAGNOLIA
- MIMOSA
- PERSIMMON
- SASSAFRAS
- SERVICEBERRY
- WILLOW
- WISTERIA
- YELLOWWOOD
- YEW
- ZELKOVA

```
R X G X Q F N X V X H U
N E Y R R E B L U M A R
K C P G S E E B K Y U L
Q P E I E L I V V C Y X
O Y P J N E D N I L Y G
L A R C H U S K T L E M
K A P O E O J V V Q O P
U P O L K H W O M F Y F
T E T S U C O L A L H B
D C P O Y M I L P K A U
M A E B N R O H L J N P
E N I P N D Y V E Y M U
```

- [ ] **HICKORY**
- [ ] **HOLLY**
- [ ] **HORNBEAM**
- [ ] **JUNIPER**
- [ ] **LARCH**
- [ ] **LINDEN**
- [ ] **LOCUST**
- [ ] **MAPLE**
- [ ] **MULBERRY**
- [ ] **OAK**
- [ ] **OLIVE**
- [ ] **PALM**
- [ ] **PECAN**
- [ ] **PINE**
- [ ] **PLUM**

```
O T U P E L O R B S C C
M O R U I E T E U Y Q J
D W B F X C S D U C O N
W N Q M J Y V W I A Y T
H S O R A L P O P M C A
I E L M A B N O K O E M
T Q C G L S G D U R Y A
E U H U V A P P L E U R
B O W J R Z S E F Q S I
E I N U S P C H N H A N
A A D P Y B S R J N Q D
M J O T A M A R A C K V
```

- ☐ ALMOND
- ☐ APPLE
- ☐ ASH
- ☐ ASPEN
- ☐ BAMBOO
- ☐ ELM
- ☐ POPLAR
- ☐ REDWOOD
- ☐ SEQUOIA
- ☐ SPRUCE
- ☐ SYCAMORE
- ☐ TAMARACK
- ☐ TAMARIND
- ☐ TUPELO
- ☐ WHITEBEAM

D	O	A	B	C	T	U	L	I	P	Y	E
O	C	C	E	D	A	R	Y	F	Z	Y	U
G	T	H	E	R	W	A	L	N	U	T	C
W	L	R	C	E	K	F	C	Z	E	C	A
O	Z	Z	H	E	Y	R	R	E	H	C	L
O	C	K	W	C	E	E	T	E	A	K	Y
D	R	O	O	W	R	B	K	Y	I	I	P
R	J	V	O	I	R	I	F	C	Z	N	T
I	U	O	D	R	R	T	B	O	U	Q	U
M	C	M	A	D	O	O	W	X	O	B	S
S	T	C	Y	P	R	E	S	S	V	O	A
L	T	U	N	T	S	E	H	C	G	V	J

- BEECH
- BEECHWOOD
- BIRCH
- BOXWOOD
- BUCKEYE
- CEDAR
- CHERRY
- CHESTNUT
- CYPRESS
- DOGWOOD
- EUCALYPTUS
- FIR
- TEAK
- TULIP
- WALNUT

N	O	G	A	R	D	P	A	N	S	C	X
D	Y	S	N	O	W	D	R	O	P	J	Z
C	Z	Y	I	V	E	R	B	E	N	A	L
R	E	W	O	L	F	L	L	E	B	B	R
W	I	A	N	A	L	P	T	Y	G	X	N
I	O	J	I	A	A	Y	I	S	Q	H	A
L	T	P	W	N	G	C	R	L	I	Q	D
L	H	S	V	E	O	L	A	A	U	H	P
O	P	E	T	M	D	G	I	C	M	T	T
W	T	E	L	O	I	V	E	L	I	A	G
C	N	L	E	N	T	O	O	B	M	A	B
W	A	U	R	E	W	O	L	F	N	U	S

☐ ACACIA ☐ BEGONIA ☐ THISTLE
☐ ALOE ☐ BELLFLOWER ☐ TULIP
☐ AMARYLLIS ☐ SNAPDRAGON ☐ VERBENA
☐ ANEMONE ☐ SNOWDROP ☐ VIOLET
☐ BAMBOO ☐ SUNFLOWER ☐ WILLOW

```
D R E R E H T A E H X U
H O L F S U C S I B I H
O Z G L Y R O M S K H T
N O F W E L K S D K Y G
E K G U O B L I D T A E
Y P K K C O E O A C C R
S J W X N H D U H G I A
U B N R L I S A L Z N N
C M Q N S P G I I B T I
K G A R D E N I A S H U
L F L O O K F E R N Y M
E S U L O I D A L G R B
```

- ☐ BLUEBELL
- ☐ DAHLIA
- ☐ DAISY
- ☐ DOGWOOD
- ☐ FERN
- ☐ FUCHSIA
- ☐ GARDENIA
- ☐ GERANIUM
- ☐ GINKGO
- ☐ GLADIOLUS
- ☐ HEATHER
- ☐ HIBISCUS
- ☐ HOLLY
- ☐ HONEYSUCKLE
- ☐ HYACINTH

```
C H A M O M I L E T Y M
C E A K E M A I R I S X
I A D J U N I P E R Z D
V H R A S C I J G Q B A
Y L A N R U R M H K F F
B L I M A T T O S G Y F
B I G L T T Y C C A M O
C L E M A T I S A U J D
U Y K C A C V O L C S I
U C Y C L A M E N D B L
W M E H T N A S Y R H C
W X B Z L A V E N D E R
```

☐ CACTUS   ☐ CLEMATIS   ☐ JASMINE

☐ CARNATION ☐ CROCUS   ☐ JUNIPER

☐ CEDAR   ☐ CYCLAMEN ☐ LAVENDER

☐ CHAMOMILE ☐ DAFFODIL ☐ LILAC

☐ CHRYSANTHEM ☐ IRIS   ☐ LILY

```
P K J U A Y W R T M Y G
W O N P E T U N I A I P
Y O I A I R E T S I W E
J O L N R E D N A E L O
A M A S S C O Y A U D N
T I A Y M E I R Y J N Y
G I N G G I T S C J O Y
B P C N N N M T S H U W
E G A S I O L O I U I B
P S V Y W Z L E S A S D
E E O D L O G I R A M X
E S O R M I R P A E J O
```

- MAGNOLIA
- MARIGOLD
- MIMOSA
- NARCISSUS
- OLEANDER
- ORCHID
- PANSY
- PEONY
- PETUNIA
- POINSETTIA
- PRIMROSE
- ROSE
- SAGE
- WISTERIA
- ZINNIA

```
B F F O N F E Y Q U E X
W B M A Y F L Y Z X P I
T S U C O L I S B U D D
G L O U S E H R E U K J
E E P V B A C Y E Y G G
S S T F T A N G T F V N
Y W P I T E D G L L L Z
A E V I M E K A E G G Y
W E U M R R G C C F K W
Y V W Q P H E D I I Z R
F I I H A H T T I R C W
X L E I T N A Q F M C I
```

- [ ] ANT
- [ ] BEETLE
- [ ] BUG
- [ ] CICADA
- [ ] CRICKET
- [ ] FIREFLY
- [ ] FLEA
- [ ] GNAT
- [ ] LOCUST
- [ ] LOUSE
- [ ] MAYFLY
- [ ] MIDGE
- [ ] TERMITE
- [ ] THRIPS
- [ ] WEEVIL

```
S D R E P P O H F A E L
I H I G B F Y B O T L R
L S D D S S T W S X E F
V S A Y Y A S I T N A M
E S M Z L T W C Q T F E
R N S D R F A F W I C A
F O E I I E N K L T U L
I W L A D H R O T Y T Y
S F F H R D P O G A T B
H L L X V W A A B A E U
K E Y Z S Y I C C Y R G
L A C E W I N G L R X D
```

- APHID
- BORER
- CADDIS
- DAMSELFLY
- DRAGONFLY
- EARWIG
- KATYDID
- LACEWING
- LEAFCUTTER
- LEAFHOPPER
- MANTIS
- MEALYBUG
- SAWFLY
- SILVERFISH
- SNOWFLEA

W	Y	B	Z	S	R	R	T	C	H	O	V
A	S	E	Y	L	F	E	N	O	T	S	V
T	P	G	H	Y	L	F	D	N	A	S	N
E	A	P	P	V	L	E	O	I	G	Q	T
R	W	H	I	T	E	F	L	Y	P	O	A
B	L	I	A	T	G	N	I	R	P	S	R
O	J	W	E	S	T	E	S	T	N	H	A
A	I	Z	G	U	B	K	N	I	T	S	N
T	P	S	N	A	K	E	F	L	Y	E	T
M	K	G	U	B	D	L	E	I	H	S	U
A	W	O	O	D	L	O	U	S	E	H	L
N	W	O	O	L	L	Y	B	E	A	R	A

- [ ] BEE
- [ ] FLY
- [ ] SANDFLY
- [ ] SHIELDBUG
- [ ] SNAKEFLY
- [ ] SPIDER
- [ ] SPRINGTAIL
- [ ] STINKBUG
- [ ] STONEFLY
- [ ] TARANTULA
- [ ] TSETSE
- [ ] WATERBOATMAN
- [ ] WHITEFLY
- [ ] WOODLOUSE
- [ ] WOOLLYBEAR

```
I L I A T W O L L A W S
X Z Y I F I R E F L Y T
Y B R L G U B F A E L I
V L U E F S P X I Z O G
E A F T R E G G I H C E
L D C N T O S H L W B R
V Y C A O E B R T W H B
E B Z L D G R P O O S E
T U E O V D A F S H M E
A G Y D Q U I R L A T T
N P D A C G P S D Y W L
T E C O C K R O A C H E
```

- BORER
- BUTTERFLY
- CADDIS
- CHIGGER
- COCKROACH
- DRAGONFLY
- FIREFLY
- HORSEFLY
- LADYBUG
- LEAFBUG
- MOTH
- SWALLOWTAIL
- TIGERBEETLE
- VELVETANT
- WASP

```
D A R T M O O R S G L T
K P T A R O K O F L J R
K L R P G U I L I N O I
O I E K O M O D O W O G
S T E T L J K J N O Z L
C V U V O A Q N O I Z A
I I L C I S N T B Y W V
U C M F V P H Q H I R B
S E O Q Z E K A K A D U
Z S A G A R M A T H A A
K B A N F F U L C S M G
O G V M I E H N U T O J
```

- BANFF
- BWINDI
- DARTMOOR
- ETOSHA
- GUILIN
- JASPER
- JOTUNHEIM
- KAKADU
- KOMODO
- KOSCIUSZKO
- PLITVICE
- SAGARMATHA
- TAROKO
- TRIGLAV
- ZION

P	I	V	K	I	L	L	A	R	N	E	Y
J	O	S	T	E	D	A	L	S	R	Z	U
K	E	I	L	A	N	E	D	W	J	J	O
I	R	J	L	R	H	P	O	S	W	J	L
N	E	S	S	A	L	W	N	S	T	Q	E
A	L	S	O	G	A	P	A	L	A	G	N
B	Q	W	N	E	L	E	U	N	O	I	Ç
A	G	N	U	R	I	V	-	C	G	O	Ó
L	F	J	O	R	D	L	A	N	D	E	I
U	R	O	T	I	M	R	U	D	D	D	S
D	O	E	D	A	L	O	E	K	I	Q	C
Z	Q	D	E	S	F	S	N	I	R	C	E

☐ DENALI ☐ FJORDLAND ☐ KILLARNEY
☐ DEOSAI ☐ GALAPAGOS ☐ KINABALU
☐ DONAU-AUEN ☐ HWANGE ☐ LASSEN
☐ DURMITOR ☐ JOSTEDALS ☐ LENÇÓIS
☐ ECRINS ☐ KEOLADEO ☐ VIRUNGA

```
N A M I B T E A C G J Y
G E E L M L E E P A S Q
U T H U A S C A R Á N T
Z X T L R K G L B L B H
N E F I A K N A L U O Y
O L A S I R O Z N E W R
L R S S X I N A H A U R
K E N A I I N E I M I S
D U A T N A L E T E N A
I Y A H N   G N O H P R
J Z S N O W D O N I A E
U L U L U N R U P G F K
```

- HUASCARÁN
- ILULISSAT
- ISALO
- KENAI
- LANTAU
- MARA
- NAMIB
- OULANKA
- PHONG NHA
- PURNULULU
- RUAHA
- RWENZORI
- SAREK
- SIMIEN
- SNOWDONIA

```
V A T N A J Ö K U L L F
P L X L W A K A T O B I Z
Z Z E M A M B O S E L I I
O R A M B K A O V A S T
V R R I E T I M E S O Y
I O E R - C A H T P W M
T N H L D P N C B I P B
I M T K A I D Y Y K K A
G J H Z R F H G T A D L
R S R L E F F B E L L O
A M U O K A Z U S T A A
Y E H C A R I V B J S H
```

- ABERDARE
- ALTYN-EMEL
- AMBOSELI
- BAIKAL
- BUFFALO
- HIDE
- TIKAL
- TSAVO
- VATNAJÖKULL
- VIRACHEY
- WAKATOBI
- YALA
- YOSEMITE
- ZAKOUMA
- ZOV TIGRA

```
R E D N U O L F A R O S
S E K X H E P K A D V P
Z E T S H S I F E U L B
X O I R Y M I F Q N T M
B Y G P A V Z F H T N C
O D B Y P D O C T Y L G
N R O O P A J H D A E R
T Q C G G P R A C T C O
X N Z H F Q U C B N B U
U M U R D I F G V K A P
X W X R M V S M R E S E
V T C Z G M C H G W S R
```

- [ ] **ANCHOVY**
- [ ] **BASS**
- [ ] **BLUEFISH**
- [ ] **CARP**
- [ ] **CATFISH**
- [ ] **COD**
- [ ] **CRAPPIE**
- [ ] **DARTER**
- [ ] **DOGFISH**
- [ ] **DRUM**
- [ ] **FLOUNDER**
- [ ] **GOBY**
- [ ] **GROUPER**
- [ ] **GRUNT**
- [ ] **GUPPY**

```
K G T T L E R E K C A M
X J N E U L A M P R E Y
X C V I L B D F Y J R M
K L L F R L I U L T F I
I Q E H A R U L J H F N
L I M H A K E M A L L N
L Y O B C D U H C H K O
I M R Q O F D U K M V W
F L A R G E M O U T H E
I K Y G F N C W C V R Z
S M O N K F I S H K R S
H S I F N O I L H E Y Q
```

- [ ] **HADDOCK**
- [ ] **HAKE**
- [ ] **HALIBUT**
- [ ] **HERRING**
- [ ] **JACK**
- [ ] **KILLIFISH**
- [ ] **LAMPREY**
- [ ] **LARGEMOUTH**
- [ ] **LING**
- [ ] **LIONFISH**
- [ ] **MACKEREL**
- [ ] **MINNOW**
- [ ] **MONKFISH**
- [ ] **MORAY**
- [ ] **MULLET**

U	H	S	I	F	K	C	O	R	A	F	B
X	G	R	D	Q	Q	C	N	O	M	J	C
W	P	O	A	M	T	U	O	P	G	X	P
D	O	A	P	C	A	J	Z	L	S	Y	U
S	A	N	D	I	S	H	C	P	L	H	O
A	J	H	A	D	C	O	N	N	H	O	U
R	H	B	S	P	L	K	S	A	H	D	P
D	E	C	U	I	M	E	E	A	R	U	V
I	F	N	R	K	F	O	F	R	U	I	E
N	N	G	V	E	O	A	P	I	E	R	P
E	C	I	A	L	P	H	M	S	S	L	Y
Y	N	E	E	D	L	E	F	I	S	H	Q

☐ NEEDLEFISH ☐ PIKE ☐ POUT
☐ OSCAR ☐ PIRANHA ☐ ROCKFISH
☐ PADDLEFISH ☐ PLAICE ☐ SARDINE
☐ PERCH ☐ POLLOCK ☐ SAURY
☐ PICKEREL ☐ POMPANO ☐ SHAD

```
G V H S I F N U S W K W
Y M Z I P C T Y V N Y H
H R E D N A Z U M H H I
C Z H S I F D R O W S T
E T A K S H U E U R U E
Z T R O V A T U F K T F
O C T E S Z R U F I L I
A O S L P D N T N T S S
H S H E E P S H E A D H
Q O S A H T A N G T Y Q
E L F C W C N N U R G A
O E S S A R W D S L J H
```

- [ ] **SHEEPSHEAD**
- [ ] **SKATE**
- [ ] **SNAPPER**
- [ ] **SOLE**
- [ ] **SPADEFISH**
- [ ] **SUNFISH**
- [ ] **SWORDFISH**
- [ ] **TANG**
- [ ] **TETRA**
- [ ] **TROUT**
- [ ] **TUNA**
- [ ] **WAHOO**
- [ ] **WHITEFISH**
- [ ] **WRASSE**
- [ ] **ZANDER**

```
C U B M B I C H O N K M
T R S E A T I G I M B Y
Z T T P L L E B T P O B
P B X O I G S P P Y X A
I R V V Y D A Z P I E X
N I L L I K I E I I R P
S A I J N E S A B V H N
C R H O P J I U S F Z W
H D P G B F P W H O E F
E W O L F H O U N D T V
R S B P S A T I K A K M
S G W E I M A R A N E R
```

☐ **AFGHAN**　☐ **BICHON**　☐ **VIZSLA**
☐ **AIDI**　☐ **BOXER**　☐ **WEIMARANER**
☐ **AKITA**　☐ **BRIARD**　☐ **WHIPPET**
☐ **BASENJI**　☐ **HUSKY**　☐ **WOLFHOUND**
☐ **BEAGLE**　☐ **TOSA**　☐ **PINSCHER**

```
F D D N U O H X O F N N
J F D N U O H Y E R G X
K Y I F U C H S B V O L
N A R T Z A I G R O C K
E A E M S N F R I S X O
O I I S C A R R T S F M
L C L T E A M I T O I O
J T V L A N D W A P N N
I U Q P O M A R N C N D
Y K S U H C L V Y J I O
A E S K I M O A A V S R
K H A R R I E R D H H P
```

- BRITTANY
- CAIRN
- CANAAN
- COLLIE
- CORGI
- DALMATIAN
- ESKIMO
- FINNISH
- FOXHOUND
- GREYHOUND
- HARRIER
- HAVANESE
- HUSKY
- KOMONDOR
- MASTIFF

```
S I O N I L A M H C H B
F P O L R M E X I C A N
T E N E T E A L U U B Z
B K P O S Z H S D H F K
O I O N L E S C T O Q T
X N I B M L T A S I O K
E G N E I A I L V N F P
R E T R N B K P A U I F
I S E G M L V I A M K P
V E R E K V J B A P M H
L A B R A D O O D L E T
N E W F O U N D L A N D
```

- BOXER
- KUVASZ
- LABRADOODLE
- LAIKA
- LEONBERGER
- MALINOIS
- MALTESE
- MASTIFF
- MEXICAN
- NEWFOUNDLAND
- PAPILLON
- PEKINGESE
- PINSCHER
- POINTER
- POODLE

X	X	T	O	E	G	Z	L	X	M	M	S
S	H	I	H	T	Z	U	R	H	P	K	T
N	R	R	I	C	I	L	P	X	X	B	A
D	E	E	E	J	X	K	M	O	S	A	B
S	E	R	L	G	R	T	U	W	E	X	Y
S	P	Y	I	I	N	E	S	L	F	N	H
S	H	A	O	H	E	I	I	H	A	T	O
X	P	E	N	M	S	W	R	R	I	S	U
Q	W	I	L	I	A	K	T	P	R	B	N
S	R	E	T	T	E	S	R	T	S	E	A
U	O	T	T	Z	I	L	M	O	O	W	T
H	A	S	U	S	S	E	X	I	Y	R	M

☐ PUG   ☐ SHELTIE   ☐ SPRINGER
☐ ROTTWEILER   ☐ SHIBA   ☐ STABYHOUN
☐ SALUKI   ☐ SHIHTZU   ☐ SUSSEX
☐ SAMOYED   ☐ SPANIEL   ☐ TERRIER
☐ SETTER   ☐ SPITZ   ☐ YORKSHIRE

```
Y C X P N O I I P R O C S
T L P A Y M G R S Z P X
J I M O W L O R E A S R
O O A D A R B O C P W Z
C N M R M M E J T G I R
O F B Z K T E E W V P V
X I A T A R A N T U L A
Y S T A I P A N A S P B
A H E B H W D K D A H L
N L C M L T W I D O W Z
X H S I F Y L L E J M W
D M E U D P C O R A L U
```

- [ ] **ADDER**
- [ ] **ASP**
- [ ] **BEE**
- [ ] **COBRA**
- [ ] **CORAL**
- [ ] **JELLYFISH**
- [ ] **KRAIT**
- [ ] **LIONFISH**
- [ ] **MAMBA**
- [ ] **SCORPION**
- [ ] **TAIPAN**
- [ ] **TARANTULA**
- [ ] **VIPER**
- [ ] **WASP**
- [ ] **WIDOW**

V	F	I	Z	O	D	O	D	O	D	L	B	M	W
C	J	V	Q	Y	F	A	C	A	N	E	C		
A	E	B	B	R	U	L	R	N	O	Q	Y		
C	P	N	B	U	L	L	E	T	N	T	J		
L	O	I	T	X	T	O	P	N	U	B	S		
H	G	N	F	I	E	K	W	D	N	V	P		
B	L	U	E	R	P	N	C	Q	S	U	U		
Q	E	D	E	D	Y	E	O	I	R	Q	F		
E	F	T	B	F	Y	U	D	R	T	C	F		
M	I	L	L	I	P	E	D	E	I	X	E		
Q	K	S	T	O	N	E	F	I	S	H	R		
S	T	I	N	G	R	A	Y	S	Z	F	C		

☐ ANT ☐ CHIRONEX ☐ PUFFER
☐ BLUE ☐ CONE ☐ STINGRAY
☐ BULLET ☐ DART ☐ STONEFISH
☐ CANE ☐ FUNNEL ☐ TICK
☐ CENTIPEDE ☐ MILLIPEDE ☐ TOAD

```
R A L L I P R E T A C W
V Z T R O V E O U K E J
H Z W E I P M Y G D Q P
L C E I V D U N G X F I
T W A S J L R B G C X R
C G Z O P D E E G B G E
J A F I R E N V V S O S
I X T C H K S A D A Z X
Z L L E W C C O K X E O
D G H R W A A O U U H W
R E T S I L B O C D R K
O E H R A G W O R M W I
```

- BLISTER
- BOX
- CATERPILLAR
- COCKROACH
- DUNG
- FIRE
- GYMPIE
- IRUKANDJI
- RAGWORM
- ROACH
- ROVE
- SEPS
- VELVET
- WEAVER
- WETA

```
D S A H C I R A T L N U
P L A T Y P U S U I Z K
Y K O L B L P W H Z X Q
R E O B A E F L E A L X
M E N D O M L E T R S H
T I T O O T A B R D H N
B A H S T M E N R I B S
F B N Z E S O N D A F D
A C L A W V F K R E W X
Q F F O U D R T N O R B
W N E D L G X A J I H T
B N I E S Y I I H R I V
```

- BOT
- CLAW
- FIREFLY
- FLEA
- HARVESTER
- HORNET
- IGUANA
- KOMODO
- LIZARD
- PLATYPUS
- SALAMANDER
- SHREW
- STONE
- TARICHA
- WARBLE

```
B Q N W K M L E M U R N
J N Z K C O C A E P V R
E W O H Z E L L E Z A G
P N T B C O W O R M I X
E O I R B U J K U S M B
U S N H E I I A O J P H
X Z H O P G G X G A A W
H N H R C L I W Z U L V
N A W S R L O T M I A A
O T T E R P A D V H P R
E O P A N D A F L I S Y
N Z P A R R O T D E R X
```

- ☐ DOLPHIN
- ☐ FALCON
- ☐ GAZELLE
- ☐ GIBBON
- ☐ HORSE
- ☐ IMPALA
- ☐ JAGUAR
- ☐ KOALA
- ☐ LEMUR
- ☐ OTTER
- ☐ PANDA
- ☐ PARROT
- ☐ PEACOCK
- ☐ SWAN
- ☐ TIGER

```
W  B  L  X  J  S  Y  H  H  X  M  D  X
Y  Q  S  A  E  Q  M  M  X  R  J  K  Q
T  A  C  B  O  B  U  V  N  Q  R  M
Q  E  D  R  A  T  I  O  G  Y  F  L
D  T  R  C  E  F  I  L  K  Y  L  J
H  C  P  G  U  V  N  N  J  K  N  X
X  O  F  D  E  R  O  O  O  X  A  L
W  H  Q  E  M  I  W  L  R  B  I  R
J  I  O  C  E  L  O  T  P  E  L  B
I  E  N  B  I  P  A  K  O  O  H  U
M  O  N  A  R  C  H  M  A  C  A  W
N  A  R  W  H  A  L  X  Y  M  O  Q
```

- ☐ BOBCAT
- ☐ BONITO
- ☐ EGRET
- ☐ HERON
- ☐ IBEX
- ☐ LYNX
- ☐ MACAW
- ☐ MAKO
- ☐ MONARCH
- ☐ NARWHAL
- ☐ OCELOT
- ☐ OKAPI
- ☐ PLOVER
- ☐ QUOKKA
- ☐ REDFOX

```
E N W S E R V A L U H F
M G A N X U A A G B R V
C V L G E P I A C E Z I
X S L E E V F W H R H C
C I A W S C A R I B O U
R O B A D A K R T K T N
Z G Y W R O E O A N G A
S U N F U I R W L D S P
D U J I M A N A T E E S
Z Q R M R J R U D U K H
Z F E E T P P O R O A T
G S M N X B S P T L Y M
```

- ☐ CARIBOU
- ☐ CHITAL
- ☐ DORADO
- ☐ GECKO
- ☐ KIWI
- ☐ KUDU
- ☐ MANATEE
- ☐ ORCA
- ☐ RAVEN
- ☐ SERVAL
- ☐ SPRING
- ☐ VICUNA
- ☐ WALLABY
- ☐ WEASEL
- ☐ XERUS

```
I I P T T A N U K I H Z
M R R V P A S R W E T Q
H V A N C M B M I Y U Z
W A T K Q Y X M J P R W
Y H I O A L L O U Q A J
L K N N A U V Y G N C T
O G A L A G S S H U O O
R G C Y Y N I I P V W Z
O U N Z D K V A F C J E
M D W O L L A F S A G B
L G V P B C E C J E K R
L K P N T F X A R I P A
```

- BONGO
- FALLOW
- GALAGO
- HAINAN
- NUMBAT
- PRATIN
- QUOLL
- SAIGA
- SIFAKA
- TANUKI
- TAPIR
- TURACO
- UAKARI
- YAK
- ZEBRA

```
S L B S S N O W D R O P O P O V
V I I H E A T H E R B U
N N A L O I D A L G X Q
O H W H A Y Y T U L I P
R H W S C C D S A S R Y
P O I N S E T T I A A N
Y Q S A I N E D R A G N
D P A E P T E E W S D P
C W P L L E W D E E P S
I N J O A I R E M U L P
Z S N A P D R A G O N K
S I T O N A H P E T S U
```

- ☐ DAISYIES
- ☐ GARDENIA
- ☐ GLADIOLA
- ☐ HEATHER
- ☐ LILAC
- ☐ PLUMERIA
- ☐ POINSETTIA
- ☐ POPPY
- ☐ ROSE
- ☐ SNAPDRAGON
- ☐ SNOWDROP
- ☐ SPEEDWELL
- ☐ STEPHANOTIS
- ☐ SWEETPEA
- ☐ TULIP

R	K	J	E	N	I	M	S	A	J	D	S
A	G	L	P	R	I	M	R	O	S	E	U
N	N	S	A	E	L	T	S	I	H	T	N
U	C	P	E	V	P	E	O	N	Y	M	F
N	S	H	E	I	E	A	H	L	L	A	L
C	A	S	Y	S	L	N	Y	Z	Y	R	O
U	A	I	M	A	O	I	D	L	F	I	W
L	L	W	N	Q	C	R	L	E	L	G	E
U	O	B	J	U	G	I	E	X	R	O	R
S	T	Z	L	A	T	S	N	B	X	L	H
M	I	M	O	S	A	E	A	T	U	D	X
O	N	G	S	R	L	I	P	E	H	T	J

- ☐ HOLLY
- ☐ HYACINTH
- ☐ IRIS
- ☐ JASMINE
- ☐ LAVENDER
- ☐ LILIES
- ☐ MARIGOLD
- ☐ MIMOSA
- ☐ PEONY
- ☐ PETUNIA
- ☐ PRIMROSE
- ☐ RANUNCULUS
- ☐ SUNFLOWER
- ☐ THISTLE
- ☐ TUBEROSE

```
R E W O L F N R O C R D
C A V A O D T G X L X A
A G I E T E Q I Z E U F
M D O A U N R K F M N F
E R L J S C A L L A I O
L L E B E U L B U T S D
L J T T Q O R C H I D I
I H S Q S M L M W S A L
A E L A Z A I N O G E B
Y B Z A G A I N N I Z Q
Q A D A N D E L I O N C
T Y A N E B R E V W X P
```

- ☐ ASTER
- ☐ AZALEA
- ☐ BEGONIA
- ☐ BLUEBELL
- ☐ CALLA
- ☐ CAMELLIA
- ☐ CLEMATIS
- ☐ CORNFLOWER
- ☐ DAFFODIL
- ☐ DANDELION
- ☐ LOTUS
- ☐ ORCHID
- ☐ VERBENA
- ☐ VIOLETS
- ☐ ZINNIA

```
Q E P O R T O I L E H C
O V N A S T U R T I U M
L G E H I B I S C U S A
E N E V O L G X O F W T
A A C R X Y H U O R I R
N I I R A A O A B D S I
D P L S O N N D D V T L
E G V O E C I A K P E L
R H E U N E U U T A R I
X D X N E G R S M N I U
P U K L F V A F T S A M
E G N I N R O M U U J L
```

- ☐ CROCUS
- ☐ DAHLIA
- ☐ FOXGLOVE
- ☐ FREESIA
- ☐ GERANIUM
- ☐ HELIOTROPE
- ☐ HIBISCUS
- ☐ LANTANA
- ☐ MAGNOLIA
- ☐ MORNING
- ☐ NASTURTIUM
- ☐ OLEANDER
- ☐ PANS
- ☐ TRILLIUM
- ☐ WISTERIA

61

B	R	G	M	Y	B	A	B	H	S	U	B
A	I	E	U	X	C	G	B	O	N	G	O
N	B	S	V	B	L	X	W	M	O	V	V
D	U	C	O	A	S	T	D	R	I	B	H
I	T	F	P	N	E	S	F	M	A	V	Y
C	T	O	X	A	B	B	A	D	G	E	R
O	E	E	G	N	O	R	U	T	N	I	B
O	R	K	R	G	N	B	A	B	O	O	N
T	F	T	Z	B	I	U	R	N	S	M	E
H	L	C	S	H	T	N	N	E	K	P	B
P	Y	G	L	N	O	U	Z	S	A	X	P
E	B	U	M	B	L	E	B	E	E	M	H

☐ BABOON   ☐ BINTURONG   ☐ BREAM
☐ BADGER   ☐ BISON   ☐ BUG
☐ BANDICOOT   ☐ BONGO   ☐ BUMBLEBEE
☐ BEAR   ☐ BONITO   ☐ BUSHBABY
☐ BEAVER   ☐ BOOBY   ☐ BUTTERFLY

```
A Z O F G Y T B W K H X
B E A G L E B A M L N K
I E T T F B E O C U P E
C F E A O P A I O B B J
H R U T G A S S A B O P
O M K Y L L I B F A O B
N B U L L E O U K T J J
L B R A N T B R Q W T K
R H J E P N G U B U O M
F H A W A C P H N E J H
D Q N V U M X W W N H O
R G M N F J W B J I Y V
```

- ☐ BASS
- ☐ BAT
- ☐ BEAGLE
- ☐ BEETLE
- ☐ BICHON
- ☐ BILLY
- ☐ BOA
- ☐ BOBCAT
- ☐ BOOBY
- ☐ BRANT
- ☐ BREAM
- ☐ BROLGA
- ☐ BUG
- ☐ BULL
- ☐ BUNNY

L	A	B	J	K	Y	L	Y	X	Z	P	J
M	H	A	G	P	O	N	L	W	T	B	X
B	A	R	R	A	M	U	N	D	I	O	Y
Z	E	T	H	E	D	G	R	E	L	N	W
Z	Z	T	N	P	B	E	M	E	L	O	Y
Q	J	T	T	A	A	O	D	U	X	B	N
D	L	P	E	A	B	Z	T	R	G	O	F
O	G	N	O	B	I	A	O	I	A	Y	B
B	U	L	L	F	R	O	G	B	N	E	F
T	Z	N	X	U	U	A	V	R	I	O	B
K	C	U	B	H	S	U	B	O	A	J	B
M	V	U	E	T	A	P	D	L	A	B	O

- BABIRUSA
- BALDPATE
- BANTAM
- BARBET
- BARRAMUNDI
- BEARDED
- BETTA
- BLENNY
- BOA
- BONGO
- BONITO
- BONOBO
- BOXER
- BULLFROG
- BUSHBUCK

```
V H K J A B U L B U L C
B D S B U R B O T J Z X
B H S I F D N A B S H Y
U B O X F I S H A U E I
D R T G X T Q V B D O V
G I N N Q G A P B Y Y B
E N O R B I B B L W D N
R D E H K C I T E U L B
I L T T U M A E R B S U
G E B U N T I N G U L V
A N B Z S A B Z F G E O
R Q M W K A B O W F I N
```

- BABBLER
- BANDFISH
- BANTENG
- BATFISH
- BIBRON
- BLUETICK
- BOUBOU
- BOWFIN
- BOXFISH
- BREAM
- BRINDLE
- BUDGERIGAR
- BULBUL
- BUNTING
- BURBOT

```
K N K G E S U O M R O D
S X P H N A M R E B O D
D X N U G N O G U D P K
O A R E T P I D N T M S
T V H U P Q H H I N M C
T D U S J M T V P Y B Z
E I H D I K D I K L Z I
R P A O O F R K E I O T
E P V R L O T K K C U D
L E V O D E E R S H P V
Y R X D I N G O A D Q H
K Y L F L E S M A D F P
```

- DAMSELFLY
- DARTFISH
- DEER
- DHOLE
- DIKDIK
- DINGO
- DIPPER
- DIPTERA
- DOBERMAN
- DOLPHIN
- DORMOUSE
- DOTTEREL
- DOVE
- DUCK
- DUGONG

```
E I S S A D S C L D D V
G O R F T R A D V A I O
P X D U I K E R Z M P K
S D D R O N G O T S P J
R Y N R E U E P B E E U
Y X Y L U H V L W L R B
D G M S U M C Z B F I K
D O N K E Y H T G L K T
B R D I S C U S I Y N J
B A P O D I D X V W D C
U H U U Z H S I F G O D
Z N E L T E E B G N U D
```

- ☐ DAMSELFLY
- ☐ DARTER
- ☐ DARTFROG
- ☐ DASSIE
- ☐ DINGY
- ☐ DIPPER
- ☐ DISCUS
- ☐ DODO
- ☐ DOGFISH
- ☐ DONKEY
- ☐ DOWITCHER
- ☐ DRONGO
- ☐ DRUM
- ☐ DUIKER
- ☐ DUNGBEETLE

```
D Q Y L F N O G A R D O
U D D D E S E R T F O X
S O A V E P I J L J G E
K G R Y R E O N I Z B J
H C W E F O R M D Z A Z
A R I I T L O M T B N X
W A N A S R Y M O S E L
K B S X M Z A I T U U V
H S I F K N O D N R S D
L L I B K C U D I G A E
Q J L Q K R A H S G O D
Z P D O N K E Y F I S H
```

- ☐ DARTER
- ☐ DARTMOOR
- ☐ DARWINS
- ☐ DAYFLYING
- ☐ DEERMOUSE
- ☐ DESERTFOX
- ☐ DOGBANE
- ☐ DOGCRAB
- ☐ DOGSHARK
- ☐ DONKEYFISH
- ☐ DONKFISH
- ☐ DRAGONFLY
- ☐ DUCKBILL
- ☐ DUSKHAWK
- ☐ DUSTMOP

N	D	C	Y	W	T	A	B	K	S	U	D
D	O	R	J	L	A	N	W	M	D	Z	J
U	N	D	A	H	F	L	A	B	Q	P	I
G	K	W	E	Z	S	Y	C	M	G	A	N
O	E	A	O	D	I	I	A	W	R	T	W
N	Y	R	R	E	I	L	F	D	E	O	A
G	R	F	X	E	E	R	W	N	O	D	D
F	A	G	X	R	S	V	T	E	W	T	Y
I	T	O	N	M	R	O	V	W	D	O	Q
S	Y	A	A	O	G	O	R	D	O	G	D
H	D	T	J	L	K	C	U	D	D	R	O
V	D	O	V	E	C	O	T	E	A	G	M

- ☐ DAYFLY
- ☐ DEERMOLE
- ☐ DEWCLAW
- ☐ DEWLIZARD
- ☐ DIRTWORM
- ☐ DOG
- ☐ DONKEYRAT
- ☐ DORMANT
- ☐ DOVECOTE
- ☐ DOWNFISH
- ☐ DROSERA
- ☐ DUCK
- ☐ DUGONGFISH
- ☐ DUSKBAT
- ☐ DWARFGOAT

```
U S D E E W K L I M I M
I F U M I Y A G R A M A
N O M J Q P T C M B A R
M B U J V S G Y A W R T
E J D M L E U A R M M E
R O S A E D X Y M G O N
G I K N T M R Z O G S G
A G I A J N X A T M E G
N M P T M B A B L D T J
S Y P E W D C M L L C M
E G E E E L P P A Y A M
R Z R M A N D R I L L M
```

- MACAW
- MAGPIE
- MAKO
- MALLARD
- MANATEE
- MANDRILL
- MANTA
- MARGAY
- MARMOSET
- MARMOT
- MARTEN
- MAYAPPLE
- MERGANSER
- MILKWEED
- MUDSKIPPER

```
M O N A R C H M E F G O
A M I C R O B A T R O N
T M Z E X M A S T I F F
D A T Y G F V K M M S F
Z M K O N I R E M E T L
M A C R O P O D C A P B
U Y K X E M M E R L I N
D F P N O E M I D Y L A
C L C K H K M I Z B C F
R Y N W H O S U D U C Z
A M E L O N Y U P G V D
B W Q S F G H I M O E Z
```

☐ MICROBAT ☐ MUDCRAB ☐ MEERKAT
☐ MERINO ☐ MASKED ☐ MEKONG
☐ MUSKOX ☐ MASTIFF ☐ MELON
☐ MACROPOD ☐ MAYFLY ☐ MERLIN
☐ MONARCH ☐ MEALYBUG ☐ MIDGE

```
X N E O T I U Q S O M E
M U S S E L O E U W S H
M U D P U P P Y U D A J
M M S R O O L D R D R S
O M E K N I M F X F C Z
T O T N M O N G R E L D
M N T M C A J T N U M D
O I A N Y M U L E Q Q W
T T E S O O G N O M Y E
M O C S G O U A C N X Z
Y R C M U S K R A T S Y
Y X Y G T E L L U M R Q
```

- ☐ MINKE
- ☐ MONGOOSE
- ☐ MONGREL
- ☐ MONITOR
- ☐ MOOSE
- ☐ MOSQUITO
- ☐ MOTMOT
- ☐ MOUSE
- ☐ MUDPUPPY
- ☐ MULE
- ☐ MULLET
- ☐ MUNTJAC
- ☐ MUSKRAT
- ☐ MUSSEL
- ☐ MYNA

```
G W B M O L E C F L T Y
E S O O G N O M W K D Q
F Y K C O S B Y L L T J
M X J C K U L G W O T P
A H O A M O O R H E N K
N L S S M U R R E L E T
T W P I S U R U L A M G
I S S N F E U Q A C A M
D G H K I K M P Q S G P
I E P U P Y L L O M G J
M O O N R A T I Q L O T
Y M U D F I S H M U T D
```

☐ MOLLY   ☐ MANTID   ☐ MOORHEN
☐ MOCCASIN   ☐ MILKFISH   ☐ MALURUS
☐ MONGOOSE   ☐ MOONRAT   ☐ MURRELET
☐ MOLE   ☐ MUDFISH   ☐ MAGGOT
☐ MACAQUE   ☐ MOORHEN   ☐

```
V X C P P E Q O G Y Q N
O Q F O R O L A S E A X
X G D P A G R D M Q Q J
P O B K W S P P O U U T
R E H T N A P I O O P E
A E N T E M K K G I P J
I N V G S E K I O L S R
R C I O U E K I P S E E
I U M F L I P A R R O T
E I B X F P N K R N R P
K V Q S D U G A O A B Z
P Y T H O N P D R U P G
```

- [ ] **PARROT**
- [ ] **PENGUIN**
- [ ] **PANTHER**
- [ ] **PUMA**
- [ ] **POODLE**
- [ ] **PUFFIN**
- [ ] **PYTHON**
- [ ] **PIGLET**
- [ ] **PIKA**
- [ ] **PRAIRIE**
- [ ] **PLOVER**
- [ ] **PIKE**
- [ ] **PORPOISE**
- [ ] **PARAKEET**
- [ ] **PRAWN**

```
P V G L L U B T I P T P
P H E A S A N T N U Q U
U N A P L A N A R I A N
G P A R R O T F I S H U
P W J C X R K P E G P M
K E G D I R T R A P I H
I C A O O L T X P T R W
S Z O F O V E K K O A X
G D E C O T M P B P N S
V B X Y A W O O U P H Y
A T Z J O E L P A Q A M
C C N I K E P O S S U M
```

- PEACOCK
- PONY
- PUG
- PELICAN
- PITBULL
- PHEASANT
- PIRANHA
- POSSUM
- PEKIN
- PARTRIDGE
- PEAFOWL
- PLANARIAN
- PATAS
- PARROTFISH
- POTOO

```
P A D E M E L O N J N K
I A E G R P Y T H O N T
K L N R O H G N O R P F
A P E T O L A D R A P V
K Y E P H P U G F I S H
Y I K L N E R N M V V Q
B R E G D I R T R A P U
D D A M Z O F Q O T F F
G D Z C X C O F J F P D
K U Z E C M P P U N W R
J C P O L E C A T P I C
S Q X M D O P U K U V V
```

- [ ] **PUGFISH**
- [ ] **POD**
- [ ] **PIKA**
- [ ] **PUFFIN**
- [ ] **PUG**
- [ ] **PARTRIDGE**
- [ ] **POLECAT**
- [ ] **POODLE**
- [ ] **PADEMELON**
- [ ] **PANTHER**
- [ ] **PARDALOTE**
- [ ] **PUKU**
- [ ] **PRONGHORN**
- [ ] **PECCARY**
- [ ] **PYTHON**

R	E	T	A	K	S	D	N	O	P	B	A
U	Z	T	E	L	T	O	R	R	A	P	B
J	F	D	P	R	E	F	F	U	P	E	K
G	J	B	Z	P	O	R	A	B	O	R	O
T	P	Y	Y	I	I	H	E	X	N	C	V
S	B	U	P	N	O	R	T	K	Y	H	X
V	Y	E	M	T	P	O	A	I	C	V	J
L	W	O	F	A	E	P	T	N	P	I	G
Y	L	Z	D	I	J	S	P	O	H	I	P
R	E	V	O	L	P	Q	L	I	P	A	P
L	X	S	M	P	A	N	G	O	L	I	N
P	T	A	R	M	I	G	A	N	T	S	I

☐ PANGOLIN ☐ PIG ☐ PONDSKATER
☐ PICKEREL ☐ PUMA ☐ PEAFOWL
☐ POTOO ☐ PIPIT ☐ PINTAIL
☐ PTARMIGAN ☐ PARROTLET ☐ PUFFER
☐ PIRANHA ☐ PLOVER ☐ PERCH

```
A F C M V K C O S S U T
L I O F E R T H H M Z U
V E J R T Z T Y Y F A R
D F L D A E H O Q I J N
B P P T N T A V M V Q I
Q Z D D S I F S L A W P
K W J H Y I R I E C T T
O A P C G Z H A R L Z O
Q H I I M I M T M H S R
M U I L L I R T K A T C
W T C R I U E M Y H T H
Z H X D T T T T U O B E F
```

- TAMARIND
- TANSY
- TARO
- TEASEL
- THISTLE
- THRIFT
- THYME
- TILIA
- TOMATO
- TORCH
- TREFOIL
- TRILLIUM
- TULIP
- TURNIP
- TUSSOCK

```
Y L I L R E G I T B L Q
K T R E E F E R N Q T T
Z M L A I S O R H P E T
G N I L I A R T K O X R
T T F P O D K V U P H I
U A I T T H I M B L E F
B X M T O A W R Q P W O
E X Y A H R R I G W J L
R I T A R O E W N I X I
O J W E N I N N E P T U
S Q G L A M X I I E U M
E T U T S A N N A A D L
```

☐ **TAMARIX** ☐ **THIMBLE** ☐ **TRAILING**
☐ **TARO** ☐ **TIGERLILY** ☐ **TREEFERN**
☐ **TARWEED** ☐ **TIGRIDIA** ☐ **TRIFOLIUM**
☐ **TEA** ☐ **TITHONIA** ☐ **TUBEROSE**
☐ **TEPHROSIA** ☐ **TORENIA** ☐ **TUTSAN**

```
M T O O T H W O R T S T S L
H K R E B U T I G E R T
S R C K A P F A E L N W
M Y T A M A R I S K Q I
Z M U I R C U E T S X N
O L L I R A M A T J E F
P T U T O R M E N T I L
J E D A L B Y A W T A O
F A E L Y S N A T G V W
K O T O U C H W O O D E
S U I L L O R T A T F R
I T E P M U R T R I U F
```

- TAMARACK
- TAMARILLO
- TAMARISK
- TANSYLEAF
- TASSEL
- TEUCRIUM
- TIGER
- TOOTHWORT
- TORMENTIL
- TOUCHWOOD
- TROLLIUS
- TRUMPET
- TUBER
- TWAYBLADE
- TWINFLOWER

```
V T N X E E R T G N U T
L T A N G L E F A Y I U
Y T I L S N G N C K C C
B R Y C L U U R I Z B K
N E R L K G L T T W U A
M A G E E S R U R R T H
Z C S B B C E A B G C O
B L P T O K O E S I I E
O E G C U I C D D S R I
G S G I W T W I O V X T
P X A L F D A O T N H S
T R A D E S C A N T I A
```

- TALLGRASS
- TANGLE
- TICKBERRY
- TICKSEED
- TOADFLAX
- TRADESCANTIA
- TREACLE
- TRIBULUS
- TUCKAHOE
- TUNG
- TUNGTREE
- TUTSAN
- TWIG
- TWINE
- TYLECODON

```
H G O H D N U O R G E U
G C N K W A H S O G X R
L N N I C G X Q S F N O
N D I I F E R K O Y Z T
E L R L F N G O B L I N
A X G A Y D E A U E S O
H S O O Z A L E U P F L
J A O D G Z R O R R E M
Z B S X D U I G G G A R
P N E X A D L G S T M X
F E U O E G A L Y E R G
T G R A S S W O R M L H
```

- ☐ GAURA
- ☐ GECKO
- ☐ GIZZARD
- ☐ GOBLIN
- ☐ GOLDFINCH
- ☐ GOOSE
- ☐ GOSHAWK
- ☐ GRASSWORM
- ☐ GRAYLING
- ☐ GREENFIN
- ☐ GREYLAG
- ☐ GROUNDHOG
- ☐ GROUPER
- ☐ GULL
- ☐

```
G R O S B E A K Z S F W
I K E Z G U A N A C O V
S U T H N O B B I G Y M
P R F I P G O E F R R O
U T A L W O T X K E J X
K D X L A D G Y N B K X
B P O T I I O R P E Y J
V Q O Q E B R G A P S T
G R I S O N R A L L U G
R I Q B M Y N E H Y C G
G T H S I F R A G G K Y
D P S A W L L A G B V U
```

- GALLWASP
- GANNET
- GARFISH
- GERBIL
- GHARIAL
- GIBBON
- GODWIT
- GOPHER
- GREBE
- GRISON
- GROSBEAK
- GUANACO
- GULL
- GUPPY

```
F A N T E V I R G H I K
D G O L D F I S H H J K D
M U S R I A F W E V W B
G V X J G C G A I B F J
R F X G L R A L R N V G
I B V U I F D G U I M Y
Z A Q R D V W I P Y G M
Z T E N E G A L A G O N
L S E A R O L A Z H T U
Y Y N R I B L A R O G R
A G O D K Y G R O U S E
G R A S S H O P A A C W
```

- [ ] **GADWALL**
- [ ] **GALAGO**
- [ ] **GENET**
- [ ] **GILA**
- [ ] **GIRAFFE**
- [ ] **GLIDER**
- [ ] **GOBY**
- [ ] **GOLDFISH**
- [ ] **GORAL**
- [ ] **GRASSHOP**
- [ ] **GRIVET**
- [ ] **GRIZZLY**
- [ ] **GROUSE**
- [ ] **GURNARD**
- [ ] **GYMNURE**

```
M G D C G G U R N A R D D
K U I D Z U U Y A G L B
X P N R G A N I S A I R
F P G V I R A D A P T X
K Y O N W A U X I G Y T
N S R H M S D B Z O X G
L A I R A H G K K O T R
J C L G G L X C X S D I
I M L G I R A F F E I S
X C A X R M H G E C K O
R E M A S S O G O L I N
U Q G L S V P I R U N Y
```

- ☐ GALAH
- ☐ GECKO
- ☐ GHARIAL
- ☐ GIRAFFE
- ☐ GOOSE
- ☐ GORILLA
- ☐ GOSSAMER
- ☐ GRISON
- ☐ GRUB
- ☐ GUAR
- ☐ GUNDI
- ☐ GUPPY
- ☐ GURNARD
- ☐ GYPSY
- ☐

```
Z G N Y D R I B G N I K
D U E H S I F I L L I K
I L A G N A K V W X L I
J W U O J A K N I K X N
M K I N G L E T H V H G
X I H K L E R T S E K F
L O J B A U W U H P S I
L P G O P A K A K U S S
U K I T T E N A L Q M H
E E D A K S I K R A W A
O K A N G A R O O O A O J
F Y F R E E D L L I K K
```

- [ ] **KAKAPO**
- [ ] **KANGAL**
- [ ] **KANGAROO**
- [ ] **KARAKUL**
- [ ] **KESTREL**
- [ ] **KILLDEER**
- [ ] **KILLIFISH**
- [ ] **KINGBIRD**
- [ ] **KINGFISH**
- [ ] **KINGLET**
- [ ] **KINKAJOU**
- [ ] **KISKADEE**
- [ ] **KITTEN**
- [ ] **KIWI**
- [ ] **KOALA**

```
D U H A F P N Q L A K V
T I J C X Y S U T R U K
Y I D P T K Z J D O E I
C E A Y K E X S K U A A
F W R R T T K L S L K K
M F H P K A W A L A T C
Y Z M J U J K V I I D U
S Y C Z M O I A D D R D
P T V B R Z K L K K O K
P A K R I Y B S A A B K
G A A L O D O M O K P N
P G V S N A Z U G A K O
```

- [ ] KAGU
- [ ] KAKA
- [ ] KAKAPO
- [ ] KALIJ
- [ ] KATYDID
- [ ] KAWALA
- [ ] KETA
- [ ] KETCH
- [ ] KODIAK
- [ ] KOMODO
- [ ] KOUPREY
- [ ] KRAIT
- [ ] KRILL
- [ ] KUDU
- [ ] KURTUS

```
K E S T R E L U D U K O
I I D H H F H H S D O W
W K G O S S K U Z Z C J
I O S J M I I O C E H X
S Z N K K R F F B W E M
X G W E A A E G L O R R
R P L E K W R K N L L X
N U A A A E S S W I I D
Z T W O P A K V T G K K
Q I X B O O O L M U O P
S N T S O R T N E K T U
K C I T O K U X L J U A
```

- KAKAPOO
- KARST
- KEKENO
- KELP
- KENTROS
- KERMODE
- KESTREL
- KILLFISH
- KINGFISH
- KIWIS
- KOB
- KOBOLD
- KOCHER
- KOTICK
- KUDU

```
N E E H Z N X K G J K H
K Y N U P K A T O B U K
O O U L U Z A W K P N M S
O L K A K A R I K I D I
K J U R K E S Q H M P A
A N J S I I D A L T A K
B L A G N A K I Y E H O
U J F K Z C M U R D S L
R K O D I A K S Y E X I
R B A Z C T X C F U M B
A A T A E S E O I V S R
L I A T B O N K B K K I
```

- KAKARIKI
- KANGAL
- KATLA
- KEDI
- KIKUYU
- KITE
- KNOBTAIL
- KODIAKS
- KOLIBRI
- KONDA
- KOOKABURRA
- KUBOTA
- KUKRI
- KUNE
- KWAZULU

```
N M E D E P I L L I M S
R M A N D R I L L Z M N
K E A N Q X S K Q G V X
Q N S N A F J Z C N J A
M Q I N T T F S F N M J
M A I L A A E I P G A M
L I L O R G N E T R A M
M I N L M A R V V S T Z
M A R N A I M E K P A I
J W C R O R N A M C Y M
Z A F A X W D K R P O R
W A Q J W T A K R E E M
```

- [ ] **MACAW**
- [ ] **MAGPIE**
- [ ] **MALLARD**
- [ ] **MANATEE**
- [ ] **MANDRILL**
- [ ] **MANTA**
- [ ] **MARE**
- [ ] **MARLIN**
- [ ] **MARTEN**
- [ ] **MASTIFF**
- [ ] **MEERKAT**
- [ ] **MERGANSER**
- [ ] **MILLIPEDE**
- [ ] **MINK**
- [ ] **MINNOW**

```
N W I T J T A R K S U M
O K T E L L U M N F I Q
D Y A Q M H H M O T M O T
P V E T M Y Y R Y A P O
Q M W K O C M A J Z O D
J J U Q N G A Y G Z D S
L H A R A O G J N R C G
E V U I R V M A T A A V
D S T A C E A E M N O M
Y A U D H T T T O J U Q
J B V O K S U L L O M M
X J F J M O O S E H E N
```

- ☐ MAGGOT
- ☐ MARGAY
- ☐ MOLE
- ☐ MOLLUSK
- ☐ MONARCH
- ☐ MONKEY
- ☐ MOOSE
- ☐ MORAY
- ☐ MOTMOT
- ☐ MOUSE
- ☐ MULLET
- ☐ MUNTJAC
- ☐ MURRE
- ☐ MUSKRAT
- ☐ MYNA

```
M D R I B G N I K C O M
I E G X V M O N I T O R
D Z I P N O D O T S A M
G N P L R A M H G V G U
E Y O A L M M E A D R S
O T P D O O A H Q W S K
X X U P O A M L Q X Z O
T H K M U L B U L K U X
U I P M A P A J L A Z V
S M Q A O L D G Q J R A
Z W C K D P A U E G V D
S U P O R C A M M M S T
```

☐ **MACROPUS** ☐ **MANX** ☐ **MOLLIE**
☐ **MAKO** ☐ **MASTODON** ☐ **MONITOR**
☐ **MALAMUTE** ☐ **MEGALODON** ☐ **MUDPUPPY**
☐ **MALLARD** ☐ **MIDGE** ☐ **MUSKOX**
☐ **MAMBA** ☐ **MOCKINGBIRD** ☐

B H Q T A N E H R O O M
M T J N E S O O G N O M
O G M Q I S Y E K N O M
U M A N U L O E Z C N A
N A R F U Y R M B V R Y
T N M W A I N A R M B F
A G O I B M R M M A V L
I A T Q D G Z A P L M Y
N B Q I B G L L U I H K
M E R I N O E L P G X V
V Y W M J B I E O G A P
H S I F D U M T G W L M

☐ MAGUARI ☐ MARMOSET ☐ MONGOOSE
☐ MALLET ☐ MARMOT ☐ MONKEY
☐ MANGABEY ☐ MAYFLY ☐ MOORHEN
☐ MANUL ☐ MERINO ☐ MOUNTAIN
☐ MARLIN ☐ MIDGE ☐ MUDFISH

C	J	Z	N	F	L	A	M	I	N	G	O
R	A	M	L	U	F	R	I	G	A	T	E
F	D	K	I	O	F	A	L	C	O	N	Y
F	O	R	K	T	A	I	L	H	W	D	G
H	C	N	I	F	Y	D	O	F	N	S	F
V	T	U	H	B	J	U	Y	D	O	F	Y
B	D	R	I	B	Y	D	O	F	T	L	N
Z	A	T	T	E	V	L	U	F	M	I	T
C	J	I	Q	N	T	N	F	I	N	C	H
F	I	N	F	O	O	T	Z	P	V	K	Z
N	I	L	O	C	N	A	R	F	B	E	W
S	F	L	Y	C	A	T	C	H	E	R	O

☐ FALCON ☐ FLYBIRD ☐ FORKTAIL
☐ FINCH ☐ FLYCATCHER ☐ FRANCOLIN
☐ FINFOOT ☐ FODY ☐ FRIGATE
☐ FLAMINGO ☐ FODYBIRD ☐ FULMAR
☐ FLICKER ☐ FODYFINCH ☐ FULVETTA

```
W U H F U R R A V E N F
A T A G E R F C Z B R U
S U O C S U F O E Z K R
H C N I F R U F W N J S
N T D H C T A C Y L F P
F I U R J F E M Q J R A
U Y G O I T U F B Y U R
R M R I M B P R Z U I R
F L J L L G E G S A T O
O F J K Z U O E E W E W
W O R C R U F R R V A F
L S I T P U L U F F T N
```

☐ FLYCATCH   ☐ FRUITEAT   ☐ FURFOWL
☐ FOWL   ☐ FULIGIN   ☐ FURRAVEN
☐ FREEBIRD   ☐ FULUPTIS   ☐ FURSPARROW
☐ FREGATA   ☐ FURCROW   ☐ FURSWAN
☐ FROGMOUTH   ☐ FURFINCH   ☐ FUSCOUS

```
X M M E R L I N M V U K
T I A A F M Y N A H T T
H N A G R E M A E O Q E
V G T N P L R W I A M H
N Z V C T I I R A N O M
E E A E C O E N U R U H
K E M O W H M F R M S M
V W A U M A R T I N E E
V L A Z F F C N O B B U
P O D R A L L A M M I P
V N N I K A N A M J R L
N E H R O O M Z B P D B
```

- ☐ MACAW
- ☐ MAGPIE
- ☐ MALLARD
- ☐ MANAKIN
- ☐ MARLIN
- ☐ MARTIN
- ☐ MERGAN
- ☐ MERLIN
- ☐ MOA
- ☐ MOORHEN
- ☐ MOTMOT
- ☐ MOUSEBIRD
- ☐ MUNIA
- ☐ MURRE
- ☐ MYNAH

```
A B L E M U R R E L E T
P N V E Z E J E A I M M
J R Y S I V A M R X O E
A V U M H P G L X M C A
Q M O N K A G F Y O K D
B M A H O K L A M N I O
W E I R O T C G M T N W
N W I N B E Y Q S E G L
I I Y I I L Z Z E Z B A
A Y T E H V E K C U I R
R A M A S K E D O M R K
F X S O M V Z T J A D J
```

- MAGPIE
- MALKOHA
- MARBLED
- MASKED
- MATIN
- MAVIS
- MEADOWLARK
- MEALY
- MELBA
- MINIVET
- MOCKINGBIRD
- MONK
- MONTEZUMA
- MURRELET
- MYNA

```
H H Y S D P L I P Y T W
B L W T Y N O E G R U S
G Q J A K O D L Q S N H
A P V R T T R U L E I O
H X M F L S S A B A E S
T S A I L F I S H H C H
D E G S R S A L M O N S
U A W H P H P A N R Y A
N W H E L O S U Z S N P
I E H S I F N U S E D L
R E P P A N S G S A R P
P D I U Q S J J E Q C K
```

☐ SAILFISH ☐ SEAWEED ☐ SPONGE
☐ SALMON ☐ SHAD ☐ SQUID
☐ SCALLOP ☐ SHRIMP ☐ STARFISH
☐ SEABASS ☐ SNAPPER ☐ SUNFISH
☐ SEAHORSE ☐ SOLE ☐ SURGEON

```
H S I F E P I N S Z U L
S N S I L V E R S I D E
T I H B X Y U X S K C Z
U P K C H Y S K C S S S
R E S A R G O W U B T W
G N S M E L T L T L F O O
E E K I R C P Y P S N R
O E G L D V S D I P E D
N L Z H L R Y D N R F F
R E Z A G R A T S A I I
X L K E T A K S T T S S
H S I F L L E W S X H H
```

- [ ] **SANDPERCH**
- [ ] **SARDINE**
- [ ] **SARGO**
- [ ] **SCULPIN**
- [ ] **SILVERSIDE**
- [ ] **SKATE**
- [ ] **SMELT**
- [ ] **SNIPE EEL**
- [ ] **SNIPEFISH**
- [ ] **SPRAT**
- [ ] **STARGAZER**
- [ ] **STONEFISH**
- [ ] **STURGEON**
- [ ] **SWELLFISH**
- [ ] **SWORDFISH**

```
U G Y F F Y H S I F D U M
W X V L L L M U S S E L K
O I D L L M O T D A M I I
Y L F Y J O E H Z I T A
Z T J I H A M - I H A M
K R Y M A N G R O V E O
P W A A A S U D E M S M
O C H N R H M A R L I N
V L S A T O S T K Z V M
R E U T B N M E D M O O
T X P E M A C K E R E L
K L T E L L U M N R P A
```

☐ MACKEREL ☐ MANGROVE ☐ MORAY
☐ MADTOM ☐ MARLIN ☐ MUDFISH
☐ MAHI-MAHI ☐ MEDUSA ☐ MULLET
☐ MAHSEER ☐ MOLA ☐ MUSSEL
☐ MANATEE ☐ MOLLY ☐

Y	Y	U	H	S	I	F	N	O	O	M	M
M	R	E	P	P	I	K	S	D	U	M	U
O	E	E	N	I	R	A	M	C	L	E	L
T	N	G	H	P	E	N	A	T	E	M	L
T	O	N	A	L	E	M	C	G	E	I	O
L	I	H	X	N	Y	K	K	A	X	C	W
E	G	Z	F	B	Y	M	E	Y	C	R	A
D	I	V	Y	M	A	C	R	O	K	O	Y
E	Q	M	Y	S	I	D	T	G	X	F	F
M	E	G	A	L	O	D	O	N	D	O	R
X	J	A	T	M	O	N	G	O	O	S	E
H	T	N	A	C	A	N	O	M	X	S	S

☐ MACKER ☐ MELANO ☐ MOONFISH
☐ MACRO ☐ METANEPH ☐ MOTTLED
☐ MARINE ☐ MICROFOSS ☐ MUDSKIPPER
☐ MEGALODON ☐ MONACANTH ☐ MULLOWAY
☐ MEGANYCT ☐ MONGOOSE ☐ MYSID

THANK YOU FOR PLAYING | HOPEFULLY YOU'VE HAD | A GOOD TIME | REVIEWS WILL BE APPRECIATED

```
X D O M J A Y H W E X L
Q T E H T F K H K R O Z
U H W T H I O R A N A V
G A J D A X M H B J S O
C N S W E I V E R T U M
I K I E I G C Y Z O W K
I F X Y V L L E D O S B
D Z V O A ' L B R O F P
L A O Y L L U F E P O H
J G H O Z C P O I B P G
M S B U U W A Y Y S U A
O O B I C V P H L T I W
```

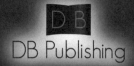

Made in United States
Troutdale, OR
01/10/2025